# MICROWAVE MUG MEALS COOKBOOK

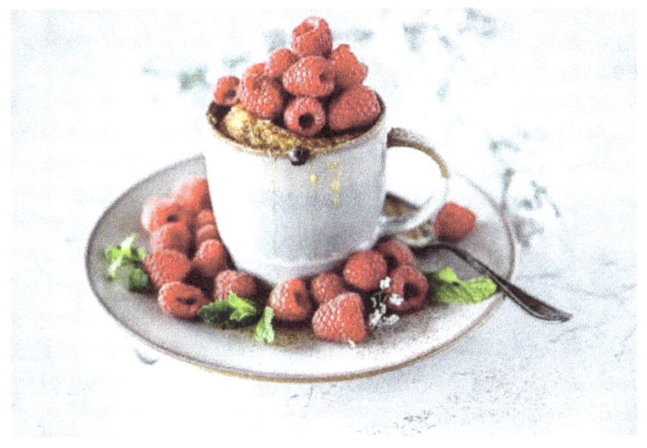

*QUICK AND EASY MICROWAVE MUG RECIPES*

*EPICUREAN KITCHEN*

# INTRODUCTION

## Why Mug Meals for Busy People?

In the hustle and bustle of modern life, time often feels like a precious commodity. Balancing work, family, and personal commitments can leave little room for elaborate meal preparation. This is where the ingenious concept of mug meals comes to the rescue. Imagine the convenience of whipping up delicious, satisfying dishes in a matter of minutes—all within the confines of a single mug. This cookbook is crafted with the busy individual in mind, offering a collection of recipes that promise to make your hectic days a bit more manageable.

Mug meals are not just a culinary trend; they are a practical solution for those who seek a harmonious blend of flavor, nutrition, and efficiency. Whether you're a student juggling classes, a professional navigating a demanding career, or a parent managing a bustling household, the simplicity and speed of mug meals can revolutionize your approach to cooking. Embrace this innovative cooking style, and you'll soon discover that it's not just about saving time—it's about savoring every moment without compromising on taste.

## Tips for Successful Mug Cooking

Embarking on the mug meal journey requires a few essential tips to ensure your culinary creations are as delightful as they are swift. Understanding the nuances of mug cooking can elevate your experience, turning each recipe into a seamless and enjoyable process. From choosing the right mug to mastering microwave techniques, we'll explore the key elements that contribute to successful mug meals. Get ready to revolutionize your kitchen routine and become a maestro of the mug.

## Essential Tools and Ingredients

Before diving into the mouthwatering recipes that await you, it's essential to familiarize yourself with the tools and ingredients that will make your mug meals a resounding success. From the ideal mug size to the must-have pantry staples, we'll guide you through setting up your mug meal kitchen. Equipping yourself with the right gear and ingredients is the first step toward creating a repertoire of quick, delicious, and satisfying mug meals that cater to your busy lifestyle. Let's ensure your mug-meal-making journey is as seamless as possible.

# DELIGHTFUL BREAKFAST RECIPES

## 1. Quick Oatmeal Mug:

- **INGREDIENTS:**
  - 1/2 cup quick oats
  - 1 cup milk (dairy or non-dairy)
  - 1 tablespoon honey or maple syrup
  - 1/2 teaspoon vanilla extract
  - Pinch of salt
- **PREP TIME:** 2 minutes
- **METHOD:**
  1. Combine oats, milk, honey, vanilla extract, and salt in a mug.
  2. Microwave for 1-2 minutes until oats are cooked and the mixture thickens.
  3. Stir well and let it cool for a minute before enjoying.

## 2. Microwave Breakfast Burrito:

- **INGREDIENTS:**
  - 1 large egg
  - 2 tablespoons diced bell peppers
  - 2 tablespoons diced tomatoes
  - 2 tablespoons shredded cheese
  - Salt and pepper to taste
  - 1 small tortilla (optional)

- **PREP TIME:** 3 minutes
- **METHOD:**

1. Whisk the egg in a mug, add bell peppers, tomatoes, cheese, salt, and pepper.

2. Microwave for 1-2 minutes, stirring halfway.

3. If desired, warm the tortilla separately, then wrap the cooked mixture in it.

# 3. Coffee Cup Quiche:

- **INGREDIENTS:**
  - 1 large egg
  - 2 tablespoons milk
  - 2 tablespoons shredded cheese
  - 1 tablespoon diced ham or cooked bacon
  - Salt and pepper to taste
- **PREP TIME:** 4 minutes
- **METHOD:**

1. In a mug, whisk together egg, milk, cheese, ham, salt, and pepper.

2. Microwave for 1.5-2 minutes, checking for doneness. Let it cool for a minute before serving.

# 4. Berry Mug Muffin:

- **INGREDIENTS:**
  - 1/4 cup flour
  - 2 tablespoons sugar
  - 1/8 teaspoon baking powder
  - Pinch of salt

- 2 tablespoons milk
- 1 tablespoon melted butter
- 1/4 cup mixed berries (fresh or frozen)
- **PREP TIME:** 5 minutes
- **METHOD:**

1. In a mug, mix flour, sugar, baking powder, and salt.
2. Add milk and melted butter, stir until smooth.
3. Gently fold in berries. Microwave for 1.5-2 minutes.

## 5. Instant Pancake Mug:

- **INGREDIENTS:**
  - 1/4 cup pancake mix
  - 2 tablespoons milk
  - 1 tablespoon maple syrup
  - 1/2 teaspoon vanilla extract
- **PREP TIME:** 3 minutes
- **METHOD:**

1. In a mug, combine pancake mix, milk, maple syrup, and vanilla extract.
2. Stir until well combined. Microwave for 1.5-2 minutes.

## 6. Yogurt Parfait in a Mug:

- **INGREDIENTS:**
  - 1/2 cup Greek yogurt
  - 1/4 cup granola
  - 2 tablespoons honey
  - 1/4 cup mixed berries
- **PREP TIME:** 2 minutes

- **METHOD:**
   1. Layer Greek yogurt, granola, honey, and berries in a mug.
   2. Repeat layers until the mug is filled. Enjoy immediately.

# 7. Peanut Butter Banana Mug Muffin:

- **INGREDIENTS:**
   - 1 ripe banana, mashed
   - 2 tablespoons peanut butter
   - 1 egg
   - 1 tablespoon honey
   - 1/4 teaspoon baking powder
- **PREP TIME:** 4 minutes
- **METHOD:**
   1. In a mug, mix mashed banana, peanut butter, egg, honey, and baking powder.
   2. Microwave for 2 minutes or until set.

# 8. Blueberry Almond Mug Cake:

- **INGREDIENTS:**
   - 1/4 cup almond flour
   - 1 tablespoon coconut flour
   - 1/4 teaspoon baking powder
   - 1 egg
   - 2 tablespoons almond milk
   - 1/4 cup blueberries
- **PREP TIME:** 5 minutes

**- METHOD:**

1. In a mug, combine almond flour, coconut flour, baking powder, egg, and almond milk.

2. Fold in blueberries. Microwave for 2-2.5 minutes.

## 9. Green Smoothie Mug:

**- INGREDIENTS:**
- 1/2 banana
- 1/2 cup spinach leaves
- 1/4 cup Greek yogurt
- 1/4 cup almond milk
- 1 tablespoon chia seeds

**- PREP TIME:** 3 minutes

**- METHOD:**

1. In a blender, combine banana, spinach, Greek yogurt, almond milk, and chia seeds.

2. Blend until smooth, then pour into a mug.

## 10. Coconut Chia Pudding Mug:

**- INGREDIENTS:**
- 2 tablespoons chia seeds    - 1/2 cup coconut milk
- 1 tablespoon honey   - 1/4 teaspoon vanilla extract

**- PREP TIME:** 5 minutes (plus chilling time)

**- METHOD:**

1. In a mug, mix chia seeds, coconut milk, honey, and vanilla extract.

2. Stir well, cover, and refrigerate for at least 2 hours or overnight.

# DELICIOUS LUNCH RECIPES

## 1. Classic Mac 'n' Cheese Mug

**INGREDIENTS:**
- 1/2 cup elbow macaroni
- 1/2 cup shredded cheddar cheese
- 1/4 cup milk
- 1/4 cup water
- 1/2 tablespoon butter
- Salt and pepper to taste

**PREP TIME:** 5 minutes

**METHOD:**

1. Combine macaroni, water, and salt in a mug.

2. Microwave for 2 minutes, stirring halfway.

3. Add cheese, milk, and butter. Stir well.

4. Microwave for an additional 1-2 minutes until the pasta is cooked and the cheese is melted.

## 2. Mediterranean Quinoa Mug Salad

**INGREDIENTS:**
- 1/4 cup quinoa, rinsed
- 1/2 cup cherry tomatoes, halved

- 1/4 cup cucumber, diced
- 2 tablespoons feta cheese, crumbled
- 1 tablespoon olive oil
- Fresh lemon juice to taste

**PREP TIME:** 5 minutes

**METHOD:**

1. Combine quinoa and water in a mug, microwave for 3 minutes.
2. Fluff quinoa with a fork, add tomatoes, cucumber, and feta.
3. Drizzle with olive oil and lemon juice. Toss gently.

## 3. Chili in a Mug

**INGREDIENTS:**

- 1/4 cup ground beef or turkey
- 2 tablespoons kidney beans, canned
- 2 tablespoons diced tomatoes
- 1/2 tablespoon chili powder
- Salt and pepper to taste

**PREP TIME:** 5 minutes

**METHOD:**

1. Cook ground meat in a mug in the microwave for 2-3 minutes.
2. Add beans, tomatoes, chili powder, salt, and pepper. Stir well.
3. Microwave for an additional 1-2 minutes until heated through.

## 4. Creamy Tomato Basil Soup

**INGREDIENTS:**

- 1/2 cup tomato soup
- 2 tablespoons heavy cream
- 1 tablespoon fresh basil, chopped

- Salt and pepper to taste
- Croutons (optional)

**PREP TIME:** 3 minutes

**METHOD:**

1. Combine tomato soup, heavy cream, basil, salt, and pepper in a mug.
2. Stir well and microwave for 2 minutes.
3. Top with croutons if desired.

## 5. Pesto Chicken Pasta Mug

**INGREDIENTS:**
- 1/2 cup cooked chicken, shredded
- 1/2 cup cooked pasta
- 2 tablespoons pesto sauce
- 1 tablespoon grated Parmesan cheese
- Cherry tomatoes for garnish

**PREP TIME:** 5 minutes

**METHOD:**

1. Layer chicken, pasta, and pesto in a mug.
2. Microwave for 2 minutes until heated.
3. Sprinkle with Parmesan and garnish with cherry tomatoes.

## 6. Teriyaki Salmon Mug

**INGREDIENTS:**
- 1/2 cup salmon fillet, cooked and flaked
- 2 tablespoons teriyaki sauce
- 1/4 cup broccoli florets, steamed
- 1/2 cup cooked white rice

**PREP TIME:** 4 minutes
**METHOD:**
1. Combine salmon, teriyaki sauce, broccoli, and rice in a mug.
2. Microwave for 2 minutes, stirring halfway.

## 7. Taco Tuesday Mug

**INGREDIENTS:**
- 1/4 cup ground beef or turkey
- 1 tablespoon taco seasoning
- 2 tablespoons black beans, canned
- 2 tablespoons corn kernels, canned
- Shredded lettuce, diced tomatoes, and cheese for topping
**PREP TIME:** 4 minutes
**METHOD:**
1. Cook ground meat with taco seasoning in a mug for 2-3 minutes.
2. Add black beans and corn, stir well.
3. Top with lettuce, tomatoes, and cheese.

## 8. BBQ Chicken and Rice Mug

**INGREDIENTS:**
- 1/2 cup cooked chicken, shredded
- 1/2 cup cooked rice
- 2 tablespoons BBQ sauce
- 1/4 cup black beans, canned
- 1/4 cup corn kernels, canned
**PREP TIME:** 5 minutes
**METHOD:** 1. Combine chicken, rice, BBQ sauce, black beans, and corn in a mug.

2. Microwave for 2 minutes, stirring halfway.

# 9. Veggie Stir-Fry in a Mug

**INGREDIENTS:**
- 1/2 cup mixed stir-fry vegetables (broccoli, bell peppers, snap peas, etc.)
- 1 tablespoon soy sauce
- 1 tablespoon sesame oil
- 1/2 cup cooked noodles or rice
**PREP TIME:** 4 minutes
**METHOD:**
1. Combine vegetables, soy sauce, and sesame oil in a mug.
2. Microwave for 2 minutes, stirring halfway.
3. Mix in cooked noodles or rice.

# 10. Shrimp Scampi Mug

**INGREDIENTS:**
- 1/2 cup cooked shrimp, peeled
- 1 tablespoon butter
- 2 tablespoons white wine
- 1 tablespoon lemon juice
- 1 tablespoon fresh parsley, chopped
- 1/2 cup cooked linguine
**PREP TIME:** 4 minutes
**METHOD:** 1. Combine shrimp, butter, white wine, lemon juice, and parsley in a mug.
2. Microwave for 2 minutes, stirring halfway.
3. Toss with cooked linguine.

# DELIGHTFUL DINNER RECIPES

## 1. Taco Tuesday Mug

- **INGREDIENTS:**
  - 1/4 cup cooked ground beef
  - 2 tablespoons black beans, drained and rinsed
  - 2 tablespoons corn kernels
  - 2 tablespoons salsa
  - 1 tablespoon shredded cheddar cheese
  - 1/2 teaspoon taco seasoning
- **PREP TIME:** 5 minutes
- **METHOD:**
  1. In a microwave-safe mug, layer the cooked ground beef, black beans, corn, salsa, and cheese.
  2. Sprinkle taco seasoning on top.
  3. Microwave on high for 1-2 minutes until cheese is melted. Stir and enjoy!

## 2. Teriyaki Salmon Mug

- **INGREDIENTS:**
  - 1/2 cup salmon fillet, cubed
  - 2 tablespoons soy sauce
  - 1 tablespoon honey
  - 1 teaspoon grated ginger

- 1 clove garlic, minced
  - 1 green onion, sliced
- **PREP TIME:** 5 minutes
- **METHOD:**
  1. In a mug, combine soy sauce, honey, ginger, and garlic.
  2. Add salmon cubes to the mixture and toss to coat.
  3. Microwave on high for 2-3 minutes until salmon is cooked.
  4. Garnish with sliced green onions and serve.

# 3. BBQ Chicken and Rice Mug

- **INGREDIENTS:**
  - 1/4 cup cooked chicken, shredded
  - 1/4 cup cooked rice
  - 2 tablespoons BBQ sauce
  - 1 tablespoon black beans, drained and rinsed
  - 1 tablespoon corn kernels
  - 1 tablespoon diced tomatoes
- **PREP TIME:** 5 minutes
- **METHOD:**
  1. In a mug, mix shredded chicken, cooked rice, BBQ sauce, black beans, corn, and diced tomatoes.
  2. Microwave on high for 1-2 minutes until heated through.
  3. Stir and enjoy your BBQ chicken and rice mug.

# 4. Veggie Stir-Fry in a Mug

- **INGREDIENTS:**
  - 1/2 cup mixed stir-fry vegetables (broccoli, bell peppers, snap peas)

- 2 tablespoons soy sauce
  - 1 tablespoon sesame oil
  - 1 clove garlic, minced
  - 1/2 teaspoon ginger, grated
  - 1/4 cup cooked noodles (rice or egg noodles)
- **PREP TIME:** 7 minutes
- **METHOD:**
  1. In a mug, combine mixed vegetables, soy sauce, sesame oil, garlic, and ginger.
  2. Microwave on high for 3-4 minutes until vegetables are tender.
  3. Stir in cooked noodles and microwave for an additional 1-2 minutes.
  4. Mix well and serve your veggie stir-fry in a mug.

# 5. Shrimp Scampi Mug

- **INGREDIENTS:**
  - 1/2 cup shrimp, peeled and deveined
  - 2 tablespoons butter
  - 1 tablespoon lemon juice
  - 1 clove garlic, minced
  - 1 tablespoon chopped parsley
  - Salt and pepper to taste
- **PREP TIME:** 5 minutes
- **METHOD:**
  1. In a mug, melt butter in the microwave.
  2. Add shrimp, lemon juice, minced garlic, chopped parsley, salt, and pepper.
  3. Microwave on high for 2-3 minutes until shrimp are pink and cooked through.
  4. Stir well and serve your shrimp scampi mug.

# 6. Mediterranean Chickpea Mug

- **INGREDIENTS:**
  - 1/2 cup canned chickpeas, drained and rinsed
  - 2 tablespoons cherry tomatoes, halved
  - 1 tablespoon feta cheese, crumbled
  - 1 tablespoon olive oil
  - 1/2 teaspoon dried oregano
  - Salt and pepper to taste
- **PREP TIME:** 5 minutes
- **METHOD:**
  1. In a mug, combine chickpeas, cherry tomatoes, feta cheese, olive oil, dried oregano, salt, and pepper.
  2. Microwave on high for 1-2 minutes until heated through.
  3. Stir and enjoy your Mediterranean chickpea mug.

# 7. Caprese Mug Skewers

- **INGREDIENTS:**
  - 1/2 cup cherry tomatoes
  - 1/4 cup mozzarella balls
  - 1 tablespoon balsamic glaze
  - Fresh basil leaves
  - Salt and pepper to taste
- **PREP TIME:** 5 minutes
- **METHOD:**
  1. Alternately thread cherry tomatoes and mozzarella balls onto a skewer or toothpick.
  2. Place the skewers in a mug.
  3. Drizzle with balsamic glaze, sprinkle with salt and pepper.

4. Microwave on high for 1 minute until mozzarella starts to melt.

5. Garnish with fresh basil and serve your Caprese mug skewers.

# 8. Asian Noodle Mug Bowl

- **INGREDIENTS:**
  - 1/2 cup cooked ramen noodles
  - 2 tablespoons soy sauce
  - 1 tablespoon sesame oil
  - 1/2 cup mixed stir-fry vegetables (carrots, broccoli, snow peas)
  - 1 green onion, sliced
- **PREP TIME:** 7 minutes
- **METHOD:**

1. In a mug, mix cooked ramen noodles, soy sauce, sesame oil, and stir-fry vegetables.

2. Microwave on high for 3-4 minutes until vegetables are tender.

3. Garnish with sliced green onions and serve your Asian noodle mug bowl.

# 9. Quinoa and Veggie Mug

- **INGREDIENTS:**
  - 1/4 cup quinoa, rinsed
  - 1/2 cup mixed vegetables (bell peppers, zucchini, cherry tomatoes)
  - 1 tablespoon olive oil
  - 1/2 teaspoon dried herbs (rosemary, thyme)
  - Salt and pepper to taste
- **PREP TIME:** 8 minutes
- **METHOD:**

1. In a mug, combine quinoa, mixed vegetables, olive oil, dried herbs, salt, and pepper.

2. Add enough water to cover the ingredients.

3. Microwave on high for 5 minutes until quinoa is cooked and vegetables are tender.

4. Stir well and let it sit for 2 minutes before serving.

# 10. Pesto Chicken Pasta Mug

**- INGREDIENTS:**
- 1/2 cup cooked chicken, shredded
- 1/4 cup cooked pasta
- 2 tablespoons pesto sauce
- 1/4 cup cherry tomatoes, halved
- 1 tablespoon grated Parmesan cheese

**- PREP TIME:** 6 minutes

**- METHOD:**

1. In a mug, mix shredded chicken, cooked pasta, pesto sauce, and cherry tomatoes.

2. Microwave on high for 2-3 minutes until heated through.

3. Sprinkle with grated Parmesan cheese before serving.

Enjoy these quick and easy dinner in a mug recipes for busy nights!

# YUMMY SNACKS AND APPETIZERS

## 1. Spinach and Artichoke Dip Mug

**INGREDIENTS:**
- 1/2 cup frozen chopped spinach, thawed and drained
- 1/4 cup canned artichoke hearts, chopped
- 1/4 cup cream cheese
- 2 tablespoons mayonnaise
- 2 tablespoons grated Parmesan cheese
- 1/4 teaspoon garlic powder
- Salt and pepper to taste

**PREP TIME:** 5 minutes

**METHOD:**

1. In a mug, mix together the cream cheese and mayonnaise until smooth.

2. Add the chopped spinach, artichoke hearts, Parmesan cheese, garlic powder, salt, and pepper. Mix well.

3. Microwave for 1-2 minutes until heated through.

4. Stir and serve with your favorite crackers or bread.

## 2. Buffalo Chicken Dip Mug

**INGREDIENTS:**
- 1/2 cup shredded cooked chicken
- 2 tablespoons cream cheese

- 1 tablespoon buffalo sauce
- 1 tablespoon ranch dressing
- 2 tablespoons shredded cheddar cheese
- Green onions for garnish (optional)

**PREP TIME:** 5 minutes

**METHOD:**

1. In a mug, combine the shredded chicken, cream cheese, buffalo sauce, and ranch dressing.

2. Microwave for 1-2 minutes until the mixture is heated through and the cream cheese is melted.

3. Top with shredded cheddar cheese and microwave for an additional 30 seconds.

4. Garnish with green onions if desired. Serve with tortilla chips or celery sticks.

# 3. Caprese Mug Skewers

**INGREDIENTS:**
- 1/2 cup cherry tomatoes, halved
- 1/4 cup fresh mozzarella balls
- 1 tablespoon balsamic glaze
- Fresh basil leaves
- Salt and pepper to taste

**PREP TIME:** 5 minutes

**METHOD:**

1. Thread cherry tomatoes and mozzarella balls onto toothpicks or small skewers.

2. Arrange the skewers in a mug.

3. Drizzle with balsamic glaze and sprinkle with salt and pepper.

4. Serve as a refreshing caprese snack.

# 4. Loaded Potato Skins in a Mug

**INGREDIENTS:**
- 1 large potato, baked and scooped
- 2 tablespoons shredded cheddar cheese
- 1 tablespoon bacon bits
- 1 tablespoon sour cream
- Chopped green onions for garnish

**PREP TIME:** 10 minutes

**METHOD:**

1. In a mug, layer the scooped potato, cheddar cheese, and bacon bits.

2. Microwave for 1-2 minutes until the cheese is melted.

3. Top with sour cream and garnish with chopped green onions.

# 5. Cheesy Nachos Mug

**INGREDIENTS:**
- 1/2 cup tortilla chips
- 1/4 cup shredded Mexican cheese blend
- 2 tablespoons black beans, drained and rinsed
- 1 tablespoon diced tomatoes
- 1 tablespoon sliced jalapeños

**PREP TIME:** 5 minutes

**METHOD:**

1. In a mug, layer half of the tortilla chips, cheese, black beans, tomatoes, and jalapeños.

2. Repeat the layers.

3. Microwave for 1-2 minutes until the cheese is melted.

4. Serve with salsa and guacamole.

# 6. Mediterranean Hummus Mug

**INGREDIENTS:**
- 1/2 cup hummus
- 2 tablespoons cherry tomatoes, halved
- 1 tablespoon Kalamata olives, sliced
- 1 tablespoon feta cheese, crumbled
- Fresh parsley for garnish

**PREP TIME:** 5 minutes

**METHOD:**
1. In a mug, spread a layer of hummus.
2. Top with cherry tomatoes, Kalamata olives, and crumbled feta cheese.
3. Garnish with fresh parsley.
4. Serve with pita chips or vegetable sticks.

# 7. BBQ Chicken Nachos Mug

**INGREDIENTS:**
- 1/2 cup tortilla chips
- 1/4 cup cooked shredded chicken
- 2 tablespoons shredded cheddar cheese
- 1 tablespoon barbecue sauce
- 1 tablespoon diced red onion
- Chopped cilantro for garnish

**PREP TIME:** 5 minutes

**METHOD:**
1. In a mug, layer half of the tortilla chips, shredded chicken, and cheddar cheese.
2. Repeat the layers.

3. Drizzle with barbecue sauce and top with diced red onion.

4. Microwave for 1-2 minutes until the cheese is melted.

5. Garnish with chopped cilantro.

## 8. Pizza Dip Mug

**INGREDIENTS:**

- 1/2 cup marinara sauce
- 1/4 cup shredded mozzarella cheese
- 1 tablespoon pepperoni slices
- 1 tablespoon black olives, sliced
- Italian seasoning for garnish

**PREP TIME:** 5 minutes

**METHOD:**

1. In a mug, layer marinara sauce, mozzarella cheese, pepperoni slices, and black olives.

2. Microwave for 1-2 minutes until the cheese is melted.

3. Garnish with Italian seasoning.

4. Serve with breadsticks or crackers.

## 9. Avocado and Black Bean Salsa Mug

**INGREDIENTS:**

- 1 avocado, diced
- 2 tablespoons black beans, drained and rinsed
- 1 tablespoon corn kernels
- 1 tablespoon red onion, finely diced
- Lime juice, to taste

- Salt and pepper, to taste
**PREP TIME:** 5 minutes
**METHOD:**

1. In a mug, combine diced avocado, black beans, corn, and red onion.
2. Squeeze lime juice over the mixture and season with salt and pepper.
3. Gently toss to combine.
4. Serve with tortilla chips.

# 10. Egg and Cheese Breakfast Mug

**INGREDIENTS:**
- 1 egg
- 2 tablespoons milk
- 2 tablespoons shredded cheddar cheese
- Salt and pepper to taste
- Chopped chives for garnish (optional)

**PREP TIME:** 5 minutes
**METHOD:**

1. In a mug, whisk together the egg, milk, shredded cheddar cheese, salt, and pepper.
2. Microwave for 1-2 minutes, stirring halfway through, until the egg is cooked and the cheese is melted.
3. Garnish with chopped chives if desired.
4. Serve as a quick and savory breakfast or snack.

These mug recipes are designed to be quick, easy, and perfect for busy individuals. Adjust quantities and ingredients based on personal preferences. Enjoy your delicious mug snacks and appetizers!

# QUICK AND EASY DESSERTS IN A MUG

## 1. Molten Chocolate Mug Cake

**INGREDIENTS:**
- 4 tablespoons all-purpose flour
- 3 tablespoons granulated sugar
- 2 tablespoons cocoa powder
- 1/8 teaspoon baking powder
- a pinch of salt
- 3 tablespoons milk
- 2 tablespoons vegetable oil
- 1/4 teaspoon vanilla extract

**PREP TIME:** 5 minutes

**METHOD:**

1. In a microwave-safe mug, whisk together flour, sugar, cocoa powder, baking powder, and salt.

2. Add milk, vegetable oil, and vanilla extract to the dry ingredients. Stir until smooth.

3. Microwave on high for 60-90 seconds until the center is just set. The cake will rise as it cooks.

4. Allow it to cool for a minute before serving. Optionally, top with whipped cream or ice cream.

# 2. Peanut Butter Mug Brownie

**INGREDIENTS:**
- 3 tablespoons all-purpose flour
- 3 tablespoons brown sugar
- 2 tablespoons cocoa powder
- a pinch of salt
- 2 tablespoons milk
- 2 tablespoons vegetable oil
- 1 tablespoon peanut butter

**PREP TIME:** 5 minutes

**METHOD:**

1. In a mug, whisk together flour, brown sugar, cocoa powder, and salt.

2. Add milk and vegetable oil to the dry ingredients. Stir until well combined.

3. Drop a spoonful of peanut butter into the center of the batter.

4. Microwave on high for 60-90 seconds until set. Allow it to cool for a minute before enjoying.

# 3. Berry Mug Cobbler

**INGREDIENTS:**
- 1/4 cup mixed berries (strawberries, blueberries, raspberries)
- 2 tablespoons granulated sugar
- 3 tablespoons all-purpose flour
- 1/4 teaspoon baking powder
- a pinch of salt
- 2 tablespoons milk
- 1 tablespoon melted butter

**PREP TIME:** 5 minutes

**METHOD:**

1. In a mug, toss the berries with sugar.

2. In a separate bowl, whisk together flour, baking powder, and salt.

3. Add milk and melted butter to the dry ingredients. Mix until just combined.

4. Pour the batter over the berries in the mug.

5. Microwave on high for 60-90 seconds. Allow it to cool slightly before digging in.

# 4. Banana Nut Mug Muffin

**INGREDIENTS:**

- 1 ripe banana, mashed
- 3 tablespoons all-purpose flour
- 2 tablespoons chopped nuts (walnuts or pecans)
- 2 tablespoons brown sugar
- 1/4 teaspoon baking powder
- a pinch of cinnamon
- 2 tablespoons milk
- 1 tablespoon melted butter

**PREP TIME:** 5 minutes

**METHOD:**

1. In a mug, combine mashed banana, flour, chopped nuts, brown sugar, baking powder, and cinnamon.

2. Add milk and melted butter to the mixture. Stir until smooth.

3. Microwave on high for 90 seconds. Allow it to cool briefly before enjoying.

# 5. Snickerdoodle Mug Cookie

**INGREDIENTS:**
- 3 tablespoons all-purpose flour
- 2 tablespoons granulated sugar
- 1/8 teaspoon baking powder
- 1/4 teaspoon cinnamon
- a pinch of salt
- 2 tablespoons milk
- 1 tablespoon melted butter
- 1/4 teaspoon vanilla extract

**PREP TIME:** 5 minutes

**METHOD:**

1. In a mug, whisk together flour, sugar, baking powder, cinnamon, and salt.

2. Add milk, melted butter, and vanilla extract to the dry ingredients. Mix until well combined.

3. Microwave on high for 60-90 seconds until set. Let it cool for a minute before indulging.

# 6. Coffee Cup Cheesecake

**INGREDIENTS:**
- 3 tablespoons cream cheese, softened
- 2 tablespoons granulated sugar
- 1/4 teaspoon vanilla extract
- 1 egg yolk
- 2 tablespoons sour cream
- 1 teaspoon all-purpose flour

**PREP TIME:** 5 minutes
**METHOD:**
1. In a mug, beat together cream cheese, sugar, and vanilla extract until smooth.
2. Add the egg yolk and mix well. Stir in sour cream and flour until combined.
3. Microwave on medium heat for 90 seconds or until set. Allow it to cool before serving.

# 7. Lemon Mug Pudding

**INGREDIENTS:**
- 3 tablespoons granulated sugar
- 2 tablespoons all-purpose flour
- a pinch of salt
- 2 tablespoons lemon juice
- 2 teaspoons lemon zest
- 3 tablespoons milk
- 1 tablespoon melted butter

**PREP TIME:** 5 minutes
**METHOD:**
1. In a mug, whisk together sugar, flour, and salt.
2. Add lemon juice, lemon zest, milk, and melted butter. Mix until smooth.
3. Microwave on high for 60-90 seconds until the pudding is set. Let it cool before serving.

# 8. Apple Pie in a Mug

**INGREDIENTS:** - 1 apple, peeled and diced

- 1 tablespoon granulated sugar
- 1/4 teaspoon cinnamon
- a pinch of nutmeg
- 2 tablespoons all-purpose flour
- 1 tablespoon rolled oats
- 1 tablespoon melted butter

**PREP TIME:** 5 minutes

**METHOD:**

1. In a mug, toss together diced apple, sugar, cinnamon, nutmeg, flour, and rolled oats.

2. Drizzle melted butter over the apple mixture. Mix until well coated.

3. Microwave on high for 2-3 minutes until the apples are tender. Allow it to cool slightly before serving.

# 9. Nutella Swirl Mug Brownie

**INGREDIENTS:**
- 3 tablespoons all-purpose flour
- 3 tablespoons granulated sugar
- 2 tablespoons cocoa powder
- a pinch of salt
- 3 tablespoons milk
- 2 tablespoons vegetable oil
- 1 tablespoon Nutella

**PREP TIME:** 5 minutes

**METHOD:**

1. In a mug, whisk together flour, sugar, cocoa powder, and salt.

2. Add milk and vegetable oil to the dry ingredients. Stir until well combined.

3. Drop spoonfuls of Nutella into the batter, and swirl with a toothpick.

4. Microwave on high for 60-90 seconds until set. Allow it to cool before enjoying.

# 10. Cinnamon Roll in a Mug

**INGREDIENTS:**
- 3 tablespoons all-purpose flour
- 2 tablespoons granulated sugar
- 1/4 teaspoon baking powder
- 1/4 teaspoon cinnamon
- a pinch of salt
- 2 tablespoons milk
- 1 tablespoon melted butter
- 1/4 teaspoon vanilla extract

**PREP TIME:** 5 minutes

**METHOD:**

1. In a mug, whisk together flour, sugar, baking powder, cinnamon, and salt.

2. Add milk, melted butter, and vanilla extract to the dry ingredients. Mix until smooth.

3. Microwave on high for 60-90 seconds until set. Drizzle with icing if desired. Allow it to cool slightly before indulging.

Enjoy these quick and delicious mug desserts!

# DRINKS / BEVERAGES

## 1. Chai Latte in a Mug

- **INGREDIENTS:**
  - 1 black tea bag
  - 1/2 cup milk
  - 1/2 cup water
  - 1 tablespoon sugar
  - 1/4 teaspoon ground cinnamon
- **PREP TIME:** 5 minutes
- **METHOD:** Steep the tea bag in boiling water, heat the milk separately, and combine with sugar and cinnamon. Mix well and enjoy!

## 2. Hot Chocolate for One

- **INGREDIENTS:**
  - 1 cup milk
  - 2 tablespoons cocoa powder
  - 2 tablespoons sugar
  - 1/4 teaspoon vanilla extract
- **PREP TIME:** 5 minutes
- **METHOD:** In a mug, mix cocoa powder and sugar. Heat milk, pour over the mixture, and stir until smooth. Add vanilla extract and enjoy.

# 3. Matcha Green Tea Mug

- **INGREDIENTS:**
  - 1 teaspoon matcha powder
  - 1 cup hot water
  - 1-2 teaspoons honey (optional)
- **PREP TIME:** 3 minutes
- **METHOD:** Whisk matcha powder into hot water until frothy. Add honey if desired. Enjoy the calming properties of matcha.

# 4. Ginger Lemon Tea

- **INGREDIENTS:**
  - 1-inch ginger, grated
  - 1 tablespoon honey
  - 1 tablespoon lemon juice
- **PREP TIME:** 5 minutes
- **METHOD:** Combine grated ginger with hot water. Add honey and lemon juice. Strain and savor the soothing tea.

# 5. Iced Coffee Delight

- **INGREDIENTS:**
  - 1/2 cup brewed coffee, chilled
  - 1/2 cup milk
  - 1 tablespoon sugar
  - Ice cubes
- **PREP TIME:** 5 minutes
- **METHOD:** Mix coffee with sugar, add milk, and stir. Pour over ice cubes and enjoy a quick iced coffee.

# 6. Turmeric Golden Milk

- **INGREDIENTS:**
  - 1 cup milk (dairy or plant-based)
  - 1/2 teaspoon ground turmeric
  - 1/4 teaspoon ground cinnamon
  - 1 teaspoon honey
- **PREP TIME:** 4 minutes
- **METHOD:** Heat milk, add turmeric and cinnamon, stir well. Sweeten with honey and enjoy the anti-inflammatory benefits.

# 7. Berry Blast Smoothie

- **INGREDIENTS:**
  - 1/2 cup mixed berries (strawberries, blueberries, raspberries)
  - 1/2 cup yogurt
  - 1/4 cup orange juice
  - 1 tablespoon honey
- **PREP TIME:** 3 minutes
- **METHOD:** Blend berries, yogurt, and orange juice until smooth. Sweeten with honey and serve chilled.

# 8. Minty Fresh Herbal Tea

- **INGREDIENTS:**
  - 1 peppermint tea bag
  - 1 cup hot water
  - 1 teaspoon honey
- **PREP TIME:** 4 minutes

- **METHOD:** Steep the tea bag in hot water, add honey, and enjoy a refreshing minty tea.

# 9. Spiced Apple Cider

- **INGREDIENTS:**
  - 1 cup apple cider
  - 1 cinnamon stick
  - 2 cloves
  - 1 slice of orange
- **PREP TIME:** 5 minutes
- **METHOD:** Heat apple cider with cinnamon stick and cloves. Squeeze in the orange slice. Strain and enjoy the warm, spiced cider.

# 10. Coconut Chai Hot Toddy

- **INGREDIENTS:**
  - 1 black tea bag
  - 1/2 cup hot water
  - 1/2 cup coconut milk
  - 1 tablespoon honey
  - 1 shot of rum (optional)
- **PREP TIME:** 6 minutes
- **METHOD:** Steep the tea bag in hot water, heat coconut milk, and mix with honey. Add a shot of rum if desired. Enjoy this tropical twist on a classic hot toddy.

# LOW CARB HEALTHY RECIPES

## 1. Microwave Egg and Vegetable Breakfast Mug

**INGREDIENTS:**
- 1 egg
- 2 tablespoons chopped bell peppers
- 2 tablespoons chopped spinach
- Salt and pepper to taste

**PREP TIME:** 5 minutes

**METHOD:**
1. In a microwave-safe mug, whisk the egg.
2. Add chopped bell peppers and spinach to the mug.
3. Season with salt and pepper.
4. Microwave on high for 1-2 minutes until the egg is set.
5. Let it cool for a minute before enjoying.

## 2. Quinoa and Black Bean Lunch Mug

**INGREDIENTS:**
- 1/4 cup quinoa
- 1/2 cup water

- 1/4 cup black beans (canned, drained, and rinsed)
- 2 tablespoons salsa
- 1 tablespoon chopped cilantro

**PREP TIME:** 8 minutes

**METHOD:**

1. Rinse quinoa and place it in a mug with water.

2. Microwave for 5 minutes.

3. Stir in black beans and salsa.

4. Microwave for an additional 2-3 minutes.

5. Garnish with chopped cilantro and serve.

# 3. Salmon and Broccoli Dinner Mug

**INGREDIENTS:**
- 3 oz. salmon fillet, cubed
- 1/2 cup broccoli florets
- 1 tablespoon olive oil
- Lemon zest
- Salt and pepper to taste

**PREP TIME:** 7 minutes

**METHOD:**

1. Place salmon and broccoli in a mug.

2. Drizzle with olive oil, add lemon zest, salt, and pepper.

3. Toss to coat evenly.

4. Microwave for 3-4 minutes or until salmon is cooked.

5. Let it sit for a minute and enjoy.

# 4. Greek Yogurt and Berry Parfait Mug

**INGREDIENTS:**
- 1/2 cup Greek yogurt
- 1/4 cup granola
- 1/4 cup mixed berries (strawberries, blueberries)

**PREP TIME:** 3 minutes

**METHOD:**
1. Layer Greek yogurt, granola, and berries in a mug.
2. Repeat the layers.
3. Serve immediately or refrigerate for later.

# 5. Mushroom and Spinach Mug Omelette

**INGREDIENTS:**
- 2 eggs
- 2 tablespoons chopped mushrooms
- 2 tablespoons chopped spinach
- 1 tablespoon feta cheese (optional)
- Salt and pepper to taste

**PREP TIME:** 5 minutes

**METHOD:**
1. Whisk eggs in a mug.
2. Stir in mushrooms, spinach, and feta.
3. Season with salt and pepper.
4. Microwave for 2-3 minutes or until set.

5. Allow it to cool slightly before serving.

# 6. Sweet Potato and Chickpea Mug Bowl

**INGREDIENTS:**
- 1/2 cup diced sweet potato
- 1/4 cup cooked chickpeas
- 1 tablespoon olive oil
- Paprika, cumin, and salt to taste

**PREP TIME:** 6 minutes

**METHOD:**
1. Toss sweet potato and chickpeas in a mug with olive oil and spices.
2. Microwave for 4-5 minutes or until sweet potato is tender.
3. Stir well and enjoy.

# 7. Tomato Basil Mug Soup

**INGREDIENTS:**
- 1 cup vegetable broth
- 1/2 cup diced tomatoes
- 2 tablespoons chopped fresh basil
- Salt and pepper to taste

**PREP TIME:** 4 minutes

**METHOD:**
1. Combine vegetable broth, tomatoes, and basil in a mug.
2. Season with salt and pepper.
3. Microwave for 3 minutes or until heated through.

4. Stir well before serving.

# 8. Avocado and Black Bean Salad Mug

**INGREDIENTS:**
- 1/2 avocado, diced
- 1/4 cup black beans (canned, drained, and rinsed)
- 1 tablespoon lime juice
- Cilantro and salt to taste

**PREP TIME:** 5 minutes

**METHOD:**
1. Mix diced avocado and black beans in a mug.
2. Drizzle with lime juice and toss.
3. Season with cilantro and salt.
4. Enjoy as a refreshing salad.

# 9. Spaghetti Squash and Tomato Mug

**INGREDIENTS:**
- 1 cup cooked spaghetti squash
- 1/2 cup diced tomatoes
- 1 tablespoon olive oil
- Garlic powder, oregano, salt, and pepper to taste

**PREP TIME:** 6 minutes

**METHOD:**
1. Combine spaghetti squash and diced tomatoes in a mug.

2. Drizzle with olive oil and season with garlic powder, oregano, salt, and pepper.

3. Microwave for 3-4 minutes or until heated through.

4. Stir well and savor the flavors.

## 10. Banana Nut Mug Muffin

**INGREDIENTS:**

- 1 ripe banana, mashed
- 2 tablespoons almond flour
- 1 tablespoon chopped nuts (walnuts or almonds)
- 1/4 teaspoon baking powder
- Dash of cinnamon

**PREP TIME:** 4 minutes

**METHOD:**

1. In a mug, mix mashed banana, almond flour, chopped nuts, baking powder, and cinnamon.

2. Microwave for 2 minutes or until the muffin is set.

3. Allow it to cool before enjoying your quick and healthy mug muffin.

## 11. Microwave Egg and Vegetable Breakfast Mug

**INGREDIENTS:**

- 1 egg
- 2 tablespoons chopped bell peppers
- 2 tablespoons chopped spinach
- Salt and pepper to taste

**PREP TIME:** 5 minutes
**METHOD:**

1. In a microwave-safe mug, whisk the egg.

2. Add chopped bell peppers and spinach to the mug.

3. Season with salt and pepper.

4. Microwave on high for 1-2 minutes until the egg is set.

5. Let it cool for a minute before enjoying.

# 12. Quinoa and Black Bean Lunch Mug

**INGREDIENTS:**
- 1/4 cup quinoa
- 1/2 cup water
- 1/4 cup black beans (canned, drained, and rinsed)
- 2 tablespoons salsa
- 1 tablespoon chopped cilantro

**PREP TIME:** 8 minutes
**METHOD:**

1. Rinse quinoa and place it in a mug with water.

2. Microwave for 5 minutes.

3. Stir in black beans and salsa.

4. Microwave for an additional 2-3 minutes.

5. Garnish with chopped cilantro and serve.

# 13. Salmon and Broccoli Dinner Mug

**INGREDIENTS:**
- 3 oz. salmon fillet, cubed
- 1/2 cup broccoli florets
- 1 tablespoon olive oil
- Lemon zest
- Salt and pepper to taste

**PREP TIME:** 7 minutes

**METHOD:**
1. Place salmon and broccoli in a mug.
2. Drizzle with olive oil, add lemon zest, salt, and pepper.
3. Toss to coat evenly.
4. Microwave for 3-4 minutes or until salmon is cooked.
5. Let it sit for a minute and enjoy.

# 14. Greek Yogurt and Berry Parfait Mug

**INGREDIENTS:**
- 1/2 cup Greek yogurt
- 1/4 cup granola
- 1/4 cup mixed berries (strawberries, blueberries)

**PREP TIME:** 3 minutes

**METHOD:**
1. Layer Greek yogurt, granola, and berries in a mug.
2. Repeat the layers.

3. Serve immediately or refrigerate for later.

# 15. Mushroom and Spinach Mug Omelette

**INGREDIENTS:**
- 2 eggs
- 2 tablespoons chopped mushrooms
- 2 tablespoons chopped spinach
- 1 tablespoon feta cheese (optional)
- Salt and pepper to taste

**PREP TIME:** 5 minutes

**METHOD:**
1. Whisk eggs in a mug.
2. Stir in mushrooms, spinach, and feta.
3. Season with salt and pepper.
4. Microwave for 2-3 minutes or until set.
5. Allow it to cool slightly before serving.

# 16. Sweet Potato and Chickpea Mug Bowl

**INGREDIENTS:**
- 1/2 cup diced sweet potato
- 1/4 cup cooked chickpeas
- 1 tablespoon olive oil
- Paprika, cumin, and salt to taste

**PREP TIME:** 6 minutes

**METHOD:**

1. Toss sweet potato and chickpeas in a mug with olive oil and spices.
2. Microwave for 4-5 minutes or until sweet potato is tender.
3. Stir well and enjoy.

## 17. Tomato Basil Mug Soup

**INGREDIENTS:**
- 1 cup vegetable broth
- 1/2 cup diced tomatoes
- 2 tablespoons chopped fresh basil
- Salt and pepper to taste

**PREP TIME:** 4 minutes

**METHOD:**

1. Combine vegetable broth, tomatoes, and basil in a mug.
2. Season with salt and pepper.
3. Microwave for 3 minutes or until heated through.
4. Stir well before serving.

## 18. Avocado and Black Bean Salad Mug

**INGREDIENTS:**
- 1/2 avocado, diced
- 1/4 cup black beans (canned, drained, and rinsed)
- 1 tablespoon lime juice
- Cilantro and salt to taste

**PREP TIME:** 5 minutes

**METHOD:**

1. Mix diced avocado and black beans in a mug.
2. Drizzle with lime juice and toss.
3. Season with cilantro and salt.
4. Enjoy as a refreshing salad.

# 19. Spaghetti Squash and Tomato Mug

**INGREDIENTS:**
- 1 cup cooked spaghetti squash
- 1/2 cup diced tomatoes
- 1 tablespoon olive oil
- Garlic powder, oregano, salt, and pepper to taste

**PREP TIME:** 6 minutes

**METHOD:**

1. Combine spaghetti squash and diced tomatoes in a mug.
2. Drizzle with olive oil and season with garlic powder, oregano, salt, and pepper.
3. Microwave for 3-4 minutes or until heated through.
4. Stir well and savor the flavors.

# 20. Banana Nut Mug Muffin

**INGREDIENTS:**
- 1 ripe banana, mashed
- 2 tablespoons almond flour
- 1 tablespoon chopped nuts (walnuts or almonds)
- 1/4 teaspoon baking powder

- Dash of cinnamon

**PREP TIME:** 4 minutes

**METHOD:**

1. In a mug, mix mashed banana, almond flour, chopped nuts, baking powder, and cinnamon.

2. Microwave for 2 minutes or until the muffin is set.

3. Allow it to cool before enjoying your quick and healthy mug muffin.

These recipes are designed for busy individuals seeking nutritious and delicious meals in a hurry. Adjustments can be made to suit personal taste preferences and dietary needs.

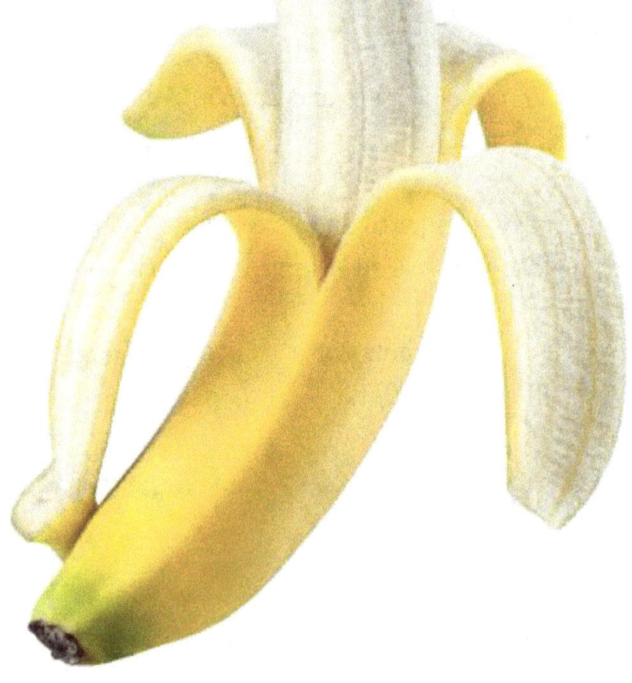

# MUG MEAL PLAN

## Day 1:

- Breakfast: Quick Oatmeal Mug
- Lunch: Classic Mac 'n' Cheese Mug
- Dinner: Teriyaki Salmon Mug
- Snack: Spinach and Artichoke Dip Mug

## Day 2:

- Breakfast: Coffee Cup Quiche
- Lunch: Mediterranean Quinoa Mug Salad
- Dinner: Taco Tuesday Mug
- Snack: Buffalo Chicken Dip Mug

## Day 3:

- Breakfast: Berry Mug Muffin
- Lunch: Chili in a Mug
- Dinner: BBQ Chicken and Rice Mug
- Snack: Caprese Mug Skewers

## Day 4:

- Breakfast: Instant Pancake Mug
- Lunch: Creamy Tomato Basil Soup

- Dinner: Veggie Stir-Fry in a Mug
- Snack: Loaded Potato Skins in a Mug

## Day 5:

- Breakfast: Pesto Chicken Pasta Mug
- Lunch: Quinoa and Veggie Mug
- Dinner: Shrimp Scampi Mug
- Snack: Mixed Berry Cobbler in a Mug

## Day 6:

- Breakfast: Mediterranean Chickpea Mug
- Lunch: Asian Noodle Mug Bowl
- Dinner: Teriyaki Salmon Mug
- Snack: Molten Chocolate Mug Cake

## Day 7:

- Breakfast: Coffee Cup Quiche
- Lunch: Greek Salad in a Mug
- Dinner: Taco Tuesday Mug
- Snack: Peanut Butter Mug Brownie

## Day 8:

- Breakfast: Berry Mug Muffin
- Lunch: Chili in a Mug
- Dinner: Veggie Stir-Fry in a Mug

- Snack: Lemon Mug Pudding

# Day 9:

- Breakfast: Quick Oatmeal Mug
- Lunch: Classic Mac 'n' Cheese Mug
- Dinner: BBQ Chicken and Rice Mug
- Snack: Spinach and Artichoke Dip Mug

# Day 10:

- Breakfast: Instant Pancake Mug
- Lunch: Creamy Tomato Basil Soup
- Dinner: Veggie Stir-Fry in a Mug
- Snack: Caprese Mug Skewers

# Day 11:

- Breakfast: Pesto Chicken Pasta Mug
- Lunch: Quinoa and Veggie Mug
- Dinner: Shrimp Scampi Mug
- Snack: Mixed Berry Cobbler in a Mug

# Day 12:

- Breakfast: Mediterranean Chickpea Mug
- Lunch: Asian Noodle Mug Bowl
- Dinner: Taco Tuesday Mug
- Snack: Molten Chocolate Mug Cake

# Day 13:

- Breakfast: Coffee Cup Quiche
- Lunch: Greek Salad in a Mug
- Dinner: Shrimp Scampi Mug
- Snack: Peanut Butter Mug Brownie

# Day 14:

- Breakfast: Berry Mug Muffin
- Lunch: Chili in a Mug
- Dinner: BBQ Chicken and Rice Mug
- Snack: Mixed Berry Cobbler in a Mug

# Day 15:

- Breakfast: Instant Pancake Mug
- Lunch: Creamy Tomato Basil Soup
- Dinner: Veggie Stir-Fry in a Mug
- Snack: Spinach and Artichoke Dip Mug

# Day 16:

- Breakfast: Coffee Cup Quiche
- Lunch: Mediterranean Quinoa Mug Salad
- Dinner: Date Night Mug Dinners
- Snack: Buffalo Chicken Dip Mug

# Day 17:

- Breakfast: Quick Oatmeal Mug
- Lunch: Classic Mac 'n' Cheese Mug
- Dinner: Festive Holiday Mug Treats
- Snack: Caprese Mug Skewers

# Day 18:

- Breakfast: Mixed Berry Cobbler in a Mug
- Lunch: Shrimp Scampi Mug
- Dinner: Teriyaki Salmon Mug
- Snack: Loaded Potato Skins in a Mug

# Day 19:

- Breakfast: Pesto Chicken Pasta Mug
- Lunch: Quinoa and Veggie Mug
- Dinner: Veggie Stir-Fry in a Mug
- Snack: Molten Chocolate Mug Cake

# Day 20:

- Breakfast: Mediterranean Chickpea Mug
- Lunch: Asian Noodle Mug Bowl
- Dinner: Taco Tuesday Mug
- Snack: Peanut Butter Mug Brownie

# Day 21:

- Breakfast: Coffee Cup Quiche
- Lunch: Greek Salad in a Mug
- Dinner: Shrimp Scampi Mug
- Snack: Lemon Mug Pudding

# Day 22:

- Breakfast: Berry Mug Muffin
- Lunch: Chili in a Mug
- Dinner: BBQ Chicken and Rice Mug
- Snack: Mixed Berry Cobbler in a Mug

# Day 23:

- Breakfast: Instant Pancake Mug
- Lunch: Creamy Tomato Basil Soup
- Dinner: Veggie Stir-Fry in a Mug
- Snack: Spinach and Artichoke Dip Mug

# Day 24:

- Breakfast: Pesto Chicken Pasta Mug
- Lunch: Quinoa and Veggie Mug
- Dinner: Shrimp Scampi Mug
- Snack: Mixed Berry Cobbler in a Mug

# Day 25:

- Breakfast: Mediterranean Chickpea Mug
- Lunch: Asian Noodle Mug Bowl
- Dinner: Teriyaki Salmon Mug
- Snack: Molten Chocolate Mug Cake

# Day 26:

- Breakfast: Coffee Cup Quiche
- Lunch: Greek Salad in a Mug
- Dinner: Taco Tuesday Mug
- Snack: Peanut Butter Mug Brownie

# Day 27:

- Breakfast: Berry Mug Muffin
- Lunch: Chili in a Mug
- Dinner: BBQ Chicken and Rice Mug
- Snack: Caprese Mug Skewers

# Day 28:

- Breakfast: Instant Pancake Mug
- Lunch: Creamy Tomato Basil Soup
- Dinner: Veggie Stir-Fry in a Mug
- Snack: Loaded Potato Skins in a Mug

# Day29:

- Breakfast: Mixed Berry Cobbler in a Mug
- Lunch: Shrimp Scampi Mug
- Dinner: Teriyaki Salmon Mug
- Snack: Spinach and Artichoke Dip Mug

# Day 30:

- Breakfast: Pesto Chicken Pasta Mug
- Lunch: Quinoa and Veggie Mug
- Dinner: Date Night Mug Dinners
- Snack: Molten Chocolate Mug Cake

# Day 31:

- Breakfast: Instant Pancake Mug
- Lunch: Creamy Tomato Basil Soup
- Dinner: Veggie Stir-Fry in a Mug
- Snack: Spinach and Artichoke Dip Mug

# Day 32:

- Breakfast: Coffee Cup Quiche
- Lunch: Mediterranean Quinoa Mug Salad
- Dinner: Date Night Mug Dinners
- Snack: Buffalo Chicken Dip Mug

# Day 33:

- Breakfast: Quick Oatmeal Mug
- Lunch: Classic Mac 'n' Cheese Mug
- Dinner: Festive Holiday Mug Treats
- Snack: Caprese Mug Skewers

# Day 34:

- Breakfast: Mixed Berry Cobbler in a Mug
- Lunch: Shrimp Scampi Mug
- Dinner: Teriyaki Salmon Mug
- Snack: Loaded Potato Skins in a Mug

# Day 35:

- Breakfast: Pesto Chicken Pasta Mug
- Lunch: Quinoa and Veggie Mug
- Dinner: Veggie Stir-Fry in a Mug
- Snack: Molten Chocolate Mug Cake

# Day 36:

- Breakfast: Mediterranean Chickpea Mug
- Lunch: Asian Noodle Mug Bowl
- Dinner: Taco Tuesday Mug
- Snack: Peanut Butter Mug Brownie

# Day 37:

- Breakfast: Coffee Cup Quiche
- Lunch: Greek Salad in a Mug
- Dinner: Shrimp Scampi Mug
- Snack: Lemon Mug Pudding

# Day 38:

- Breakfast: Berry Mug Muffin
- Lunch: Chili in a Mug
- Dinner: BBQ Chicken and Rice Mug
- Snack: Mixed Berry Cobbler in a Mug

# Day 39:

- Breakfast: Instant Pancake Mug
- Lunch: Creamy Tomato Basil Soup
- Dinner: Veggie Stir-Fry in a Mug
- Snack: Spinach and Artichoke Dip Mug

# Day 40:

- Breakfast: Coffee Cup Quiche
- Lunch: Mediterranean Quinoa Mug Salad
- Dinner: Date Night Mug Dinners
- Snack: Buffalo Chicken Dip Mug

# Day 41:

- Breakfast: Quick Oatmeal Mug
- Lunch: Classic Mac 'n' Cheese Mug
- Dinner: Festive Holiday Mug Treats
- Snack: Caprese Mug Skewers

# Day 42:

- Breakfast: Mixed Berry Cobbler in a Mug
- Lunch: Shrimp Scampi Mug
- Dinner: Teriyaki Salmon Mug
- Snack: Loaded Potato Skins in a Mug

# Day 43:

- Breakfast: Pesto Chicken Pasta Mug
- Lunch: Quinoa and Veggie Mug
- Dinner: Veggie Stir-Fry in a Mug
- Snack: Molten Chocolate Mug Cake

# Day 44:

- Breakfast: Mediterranean Chickpea Mug
- Lunch: Asian Noodle Mug Bowl
- Dinner: Taco Tuesday Mug
- Snack: Peanut Butter Mug Brownie

# Day 45:

- Breakfast: Coffee Cup Quiche
- Lunch: Greek Salad in a Mug
- Dinner: Shrimp Scampi Mug
- Snack: Lemon Mug Pudding

# Day 46:

- Breakfast: Berry Mug Muffin
- Lunch: Chili in a Mug
- Dinner: BBQ Chicken and Rice Mug
- Snack: Mixed Berry Cobbler in a Mug

# Day 47:

- Breakfast: Instant Pancake Mug
- Lunch: Creamy Tomato Basil Soup
- Dinner: Veggie Stir-Fry in a Mug
- Snack: Spinach and Artichoke Dip Mug

# Day 48:

- Breakfast: Coffee Cup Quiche
- Lunch: Mediterranean Quinoa Mug Salad
- Dinner: Date Night Mug Dinners
- Snack: Buffalo Chicken Dip Mug

# Day 49:

- Breakfast: Quick Oatmeal Mug
- Lunch: Classic Mac 'n' Cheese Mug
- Dinner: Festive Holiday Mug Treats
- Snack: Caprese Mug Skewers

# Day 50:

- Breakfast: Mixed Berry Cobbler in a Mug
- Lunch: Shrimp Scampi Mug
- Dinner: Teriyaki Salmon Mug
- Snack: Loaded Potato Skins in a Mug

# Day 51:

- Breakfast: Pesto Chicken Pasta Mug
- Lunch: Quinoa and Veggie Mug
- Dinner: Veggie Stir-Fry in a Mug
- Snack: Molten Chocolate Mug Cake

# Day 52:

- Breakfast: Mediterranean Chickpea Mug
- Lunch: Asian Noodle Mug Bowl
- Dinner: Taco Tuesday Mug
- Snack: Peanut Butter Mug Brownie

# Day 53:

- Breakfast: Coffee Cup Quiche
- Lunch: Greek Salad in a Mug
- Dinner: Shrimp Scampi Mug
- Snack: Lemon Mug Pudding

# Day 54:

- Breakfast: Berry Mug Muffin
- Lunch: Chili in a Mug
- Dinner: BBQ Chicken and Rice Mug
- Snack: Mixed Berry Cobbler in a Mug

# Day 55:

- Breakfast: Instant Pancake Mug
- Lunch: Creamy Tomato Basil Soup
- Dinner: Veggie Stir-Fry in a Mug
- Snack: Spinach and Artichoke Dip Mug

# Day 56:

- Breakfast: Coffee Cup Quiche
- Lunch: Mediterranean Quinoa Mug Salad
- Dinner: Date Night Mug Dinners
- Snack: Buffalo Chicken Dip Mug

# Day 57:

- Breakfast: Quick Oatmeal Mug
- Lunch: Classic Mac 'n' Cheese Mug
- Dinner: Festive Holiday Mug Treats
- Snack: Caprese Mug Skewers

# Day 58:

- Breakfast: Mixed Berry Cobbler in a Mug
- Lunch: Shrimp Scampi Mug
- Dinner: Teriyaki Salmon Mug
- Snack: Loaded Potato Skins in a Mug

# Day 59:

- Breakfast: Pesto Chicken Pasta Mug
- Lunch: Quinoa and Veggie Mug
- Dinner: Veggie Stir-Fry in a Mug
- Snack: Molten Chocolate Mug Cake

# Day 60:

- Breakfast: Mediterranean Chickpea Mug
- Lunch: Asian Noodle Mug Bowl
- Dinner: Taco Tuesday Mug
- Snack: Peanut Butter Mug Brownie

Congratulations on completing the "Mug Magic" 60-day meal plan! This journey has empowered you with a wealth of quick, delicious, and convenient mug meals. Continue to explore new recipes and savor the magic of mug cooking!

# Conclusion: Embracing the Mug Meal Lifestyle

Congratulations on completing your journey through the world of mug meals designed for busy people! In this cookbook, we've explored the art of creating delicious, time-saving dishes that fit seamlessly into the fast-paced rhythm of your life.

As you've discovered, mug meals are not just a quick fix but a culinary adventure that allows you to savor diverse flavors without compromising your precious time. Whether you're a busy professional, a student racing against deadlines, or a parent juggling multiple responsibilities, these recipes were crafted with you in mind.

In the final chapter, let's reflect on the key takeaways and the benefits of embracing the mug meal lifestyle:

## 1. Time Efficiency: 
Mug meals are your secret weapon when time is of the essence. With minimal prep and speedy cook times, you can enjoy a hot and satisfying meal in minutes, freeing up more time for what matters most.

## 2. Culinary Creativity: 
The mug is not just a vessel; it's a canvas for culinary expression. From breakfast to dessert, these recipes showcase the versatility of mug cooking, encouraging you to experiment with flavors, textures, and ingredients.

## 3. Portion Control: 
Mug meals are inherently portion-controlled, helping you maintain a balanced and mindful

approach to your diet. No more leftovers lingering in the fridge—each mug contains a perfectly portioned serving.

## 4. Minimal Clean up: Say goodbye to piles of dirty dishes. With mug meals, you can whip up a delightful dish using just a mug and a few utensils, minimizing the time spent on clean up and maximizing the time spent enjoying your meal.

## 5. Share the Joy: The simplicity and convenience of mug meals make them ideal for sharing. Host a mug meal party, invite friends over for a mug brunch, or surprise your loved ones with a thoughtful mug treat. These recipes are meant to be shared and enjoyed together.

Thank you for taking this flavorful journey with us. May your mug always be filled with delicious possibilities, and may each bite bring a moment of joy and satisfaction to your busy life. Happy mug cooking!